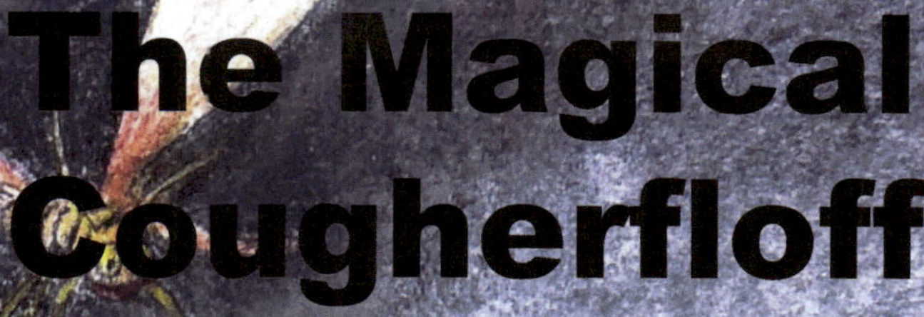

The Magical Cougherfloff

By
Owen Tong

Inspired by, and dedicated to my grandson Seth, the poorly child in the story. Credit to Robert Austin for the original Artwork.

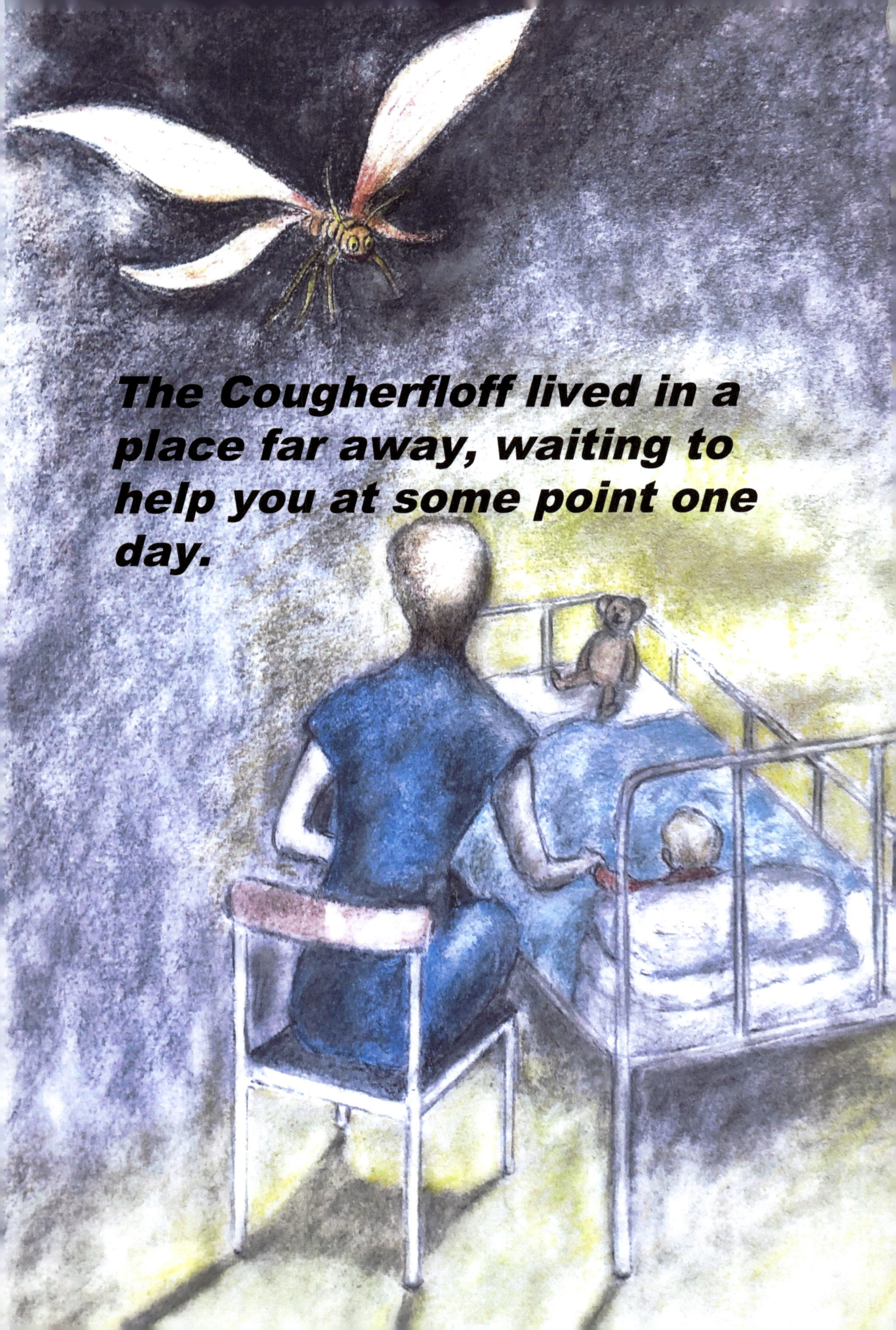

The Cougherfloff lived in a place far away, waiting to help you at some point one day.

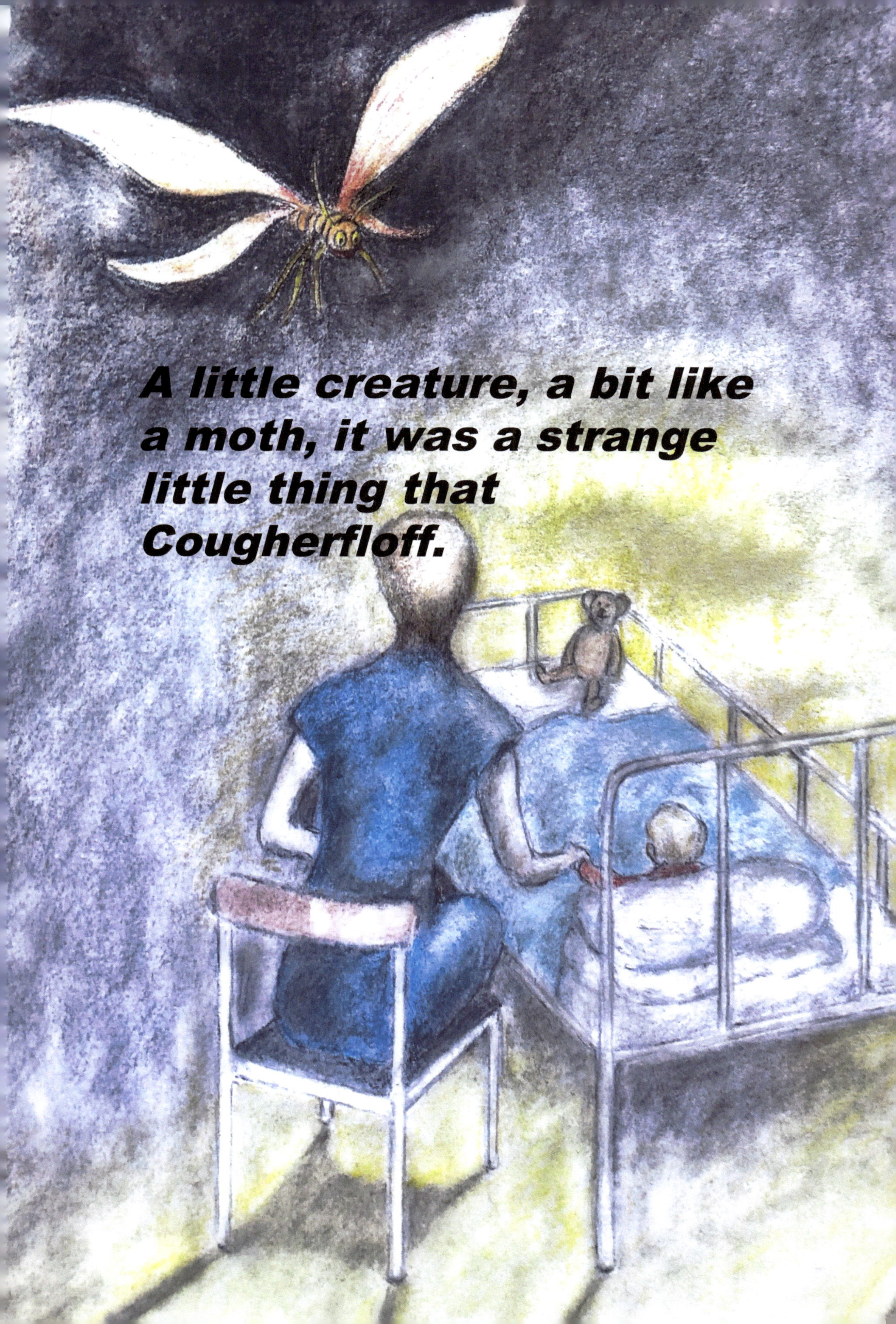

A little creature, a bit like a moth, it was a strange little thing that Cougherfloff.

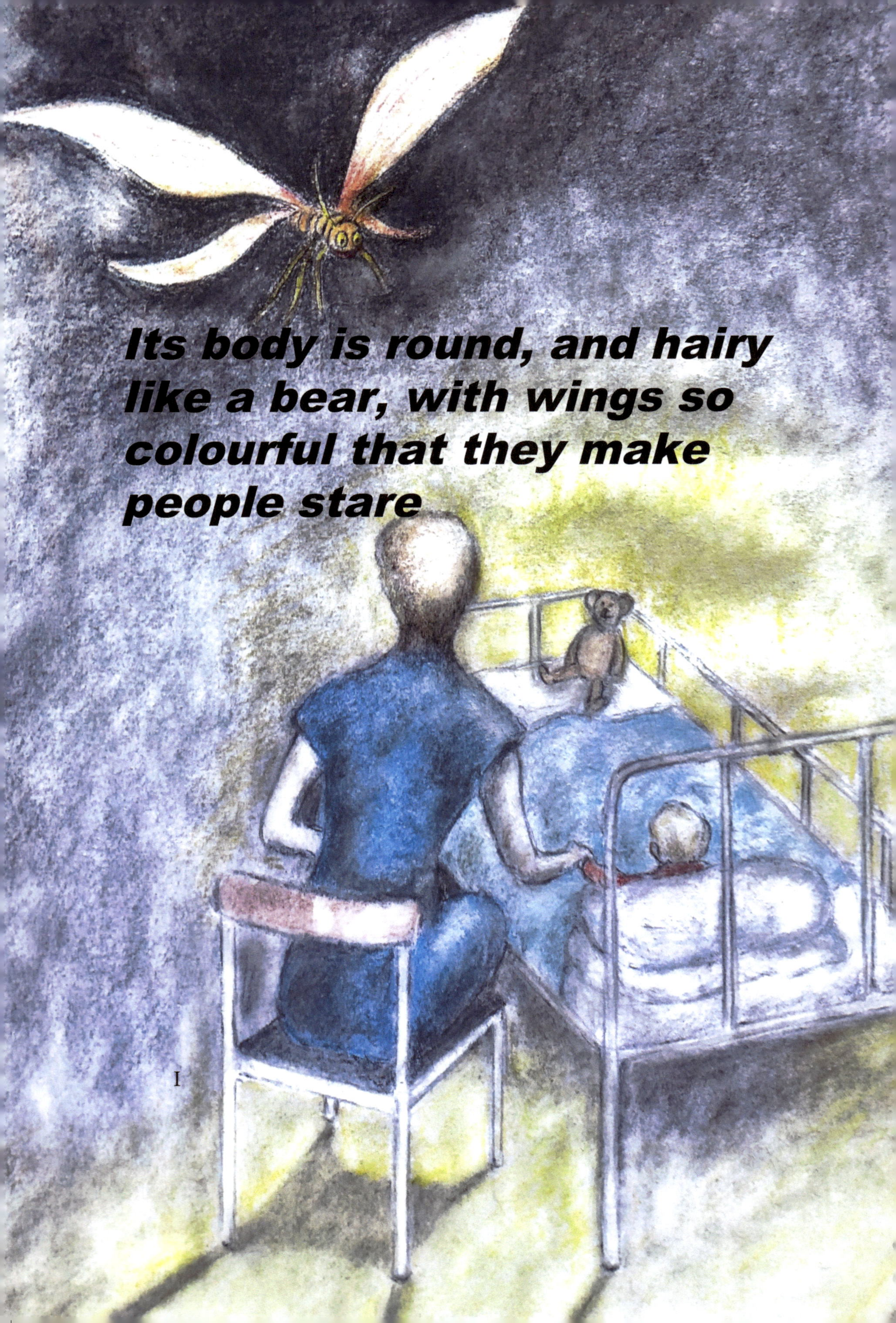
Its body is round, and hairy like a bear, with wings so colourful that they make people stare

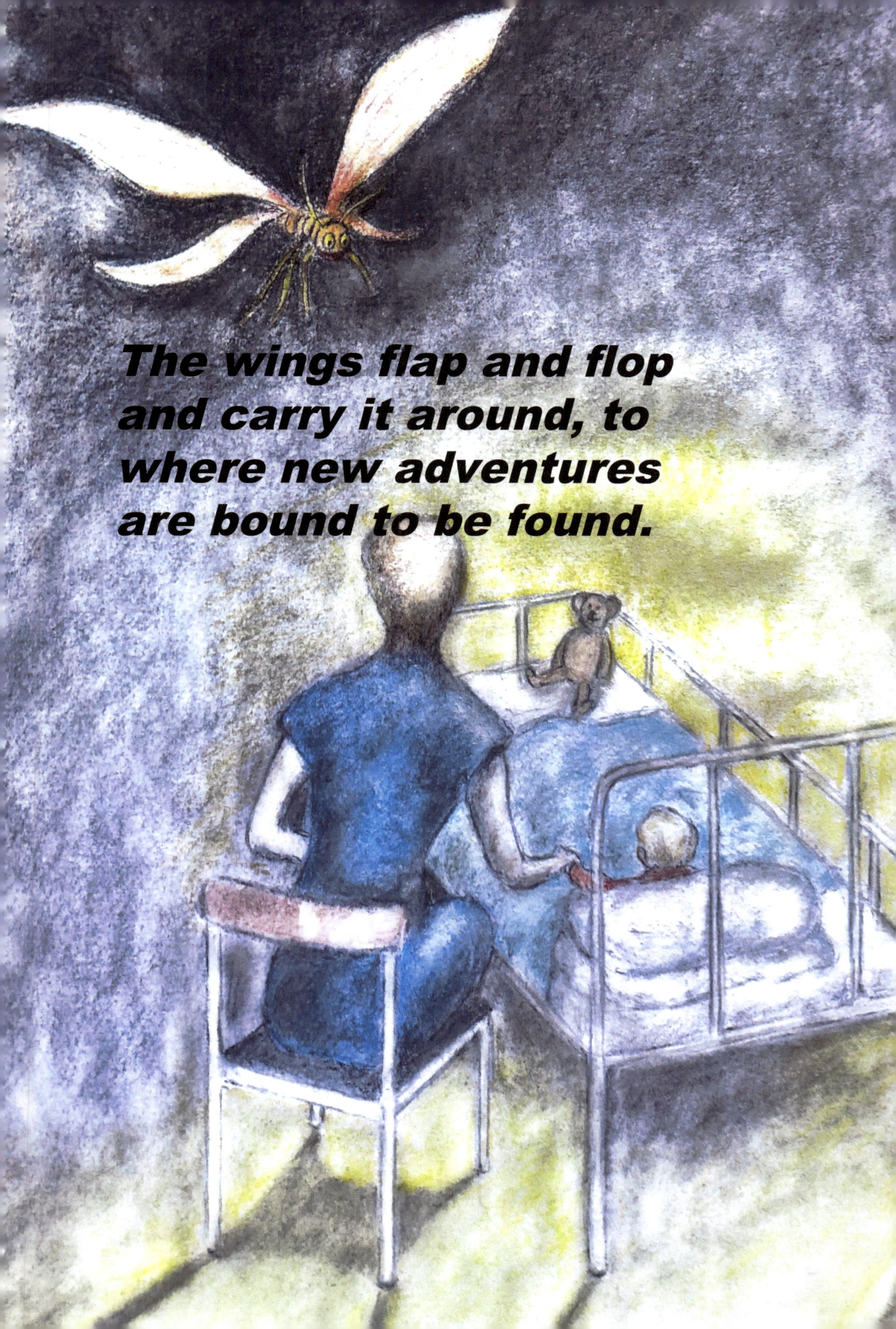
The wings flap and flop
and carry it around, to
where new adventures
are bound to be found.

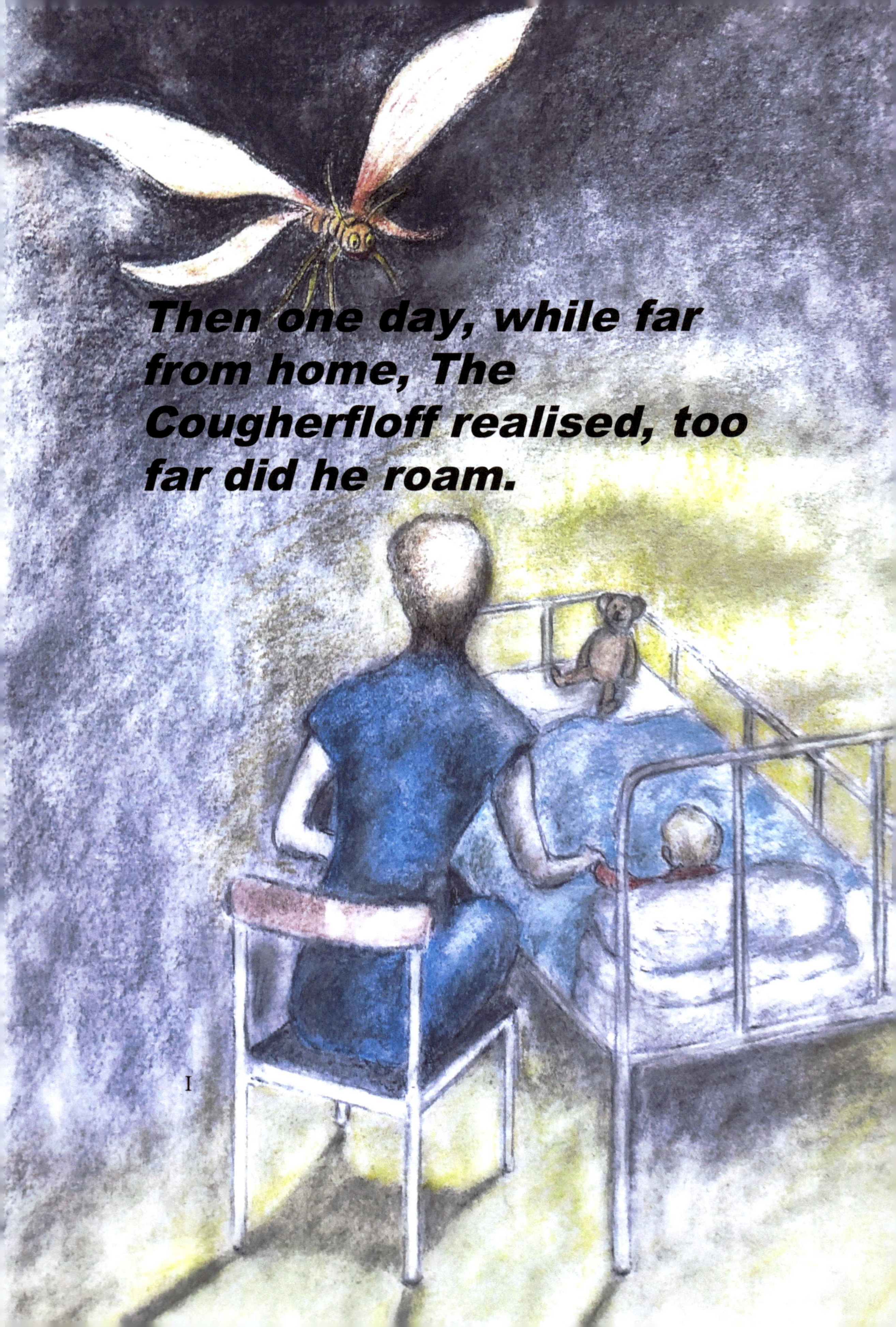
Then one day, while far from home, The Cougherfloff realised, too far did he roam.

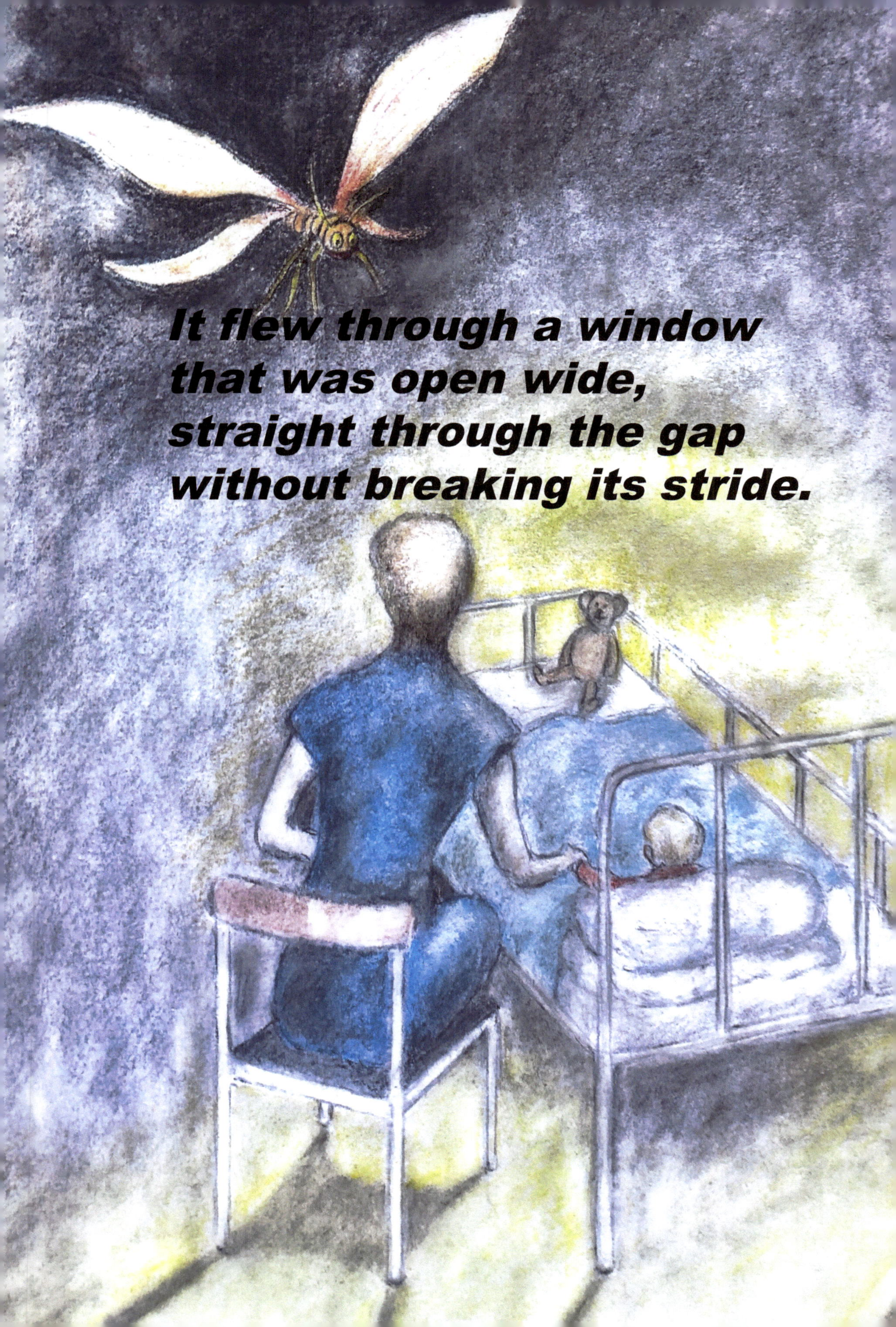
It flew through a window
that was open wide,
straight through the gap
without breaking its stride.

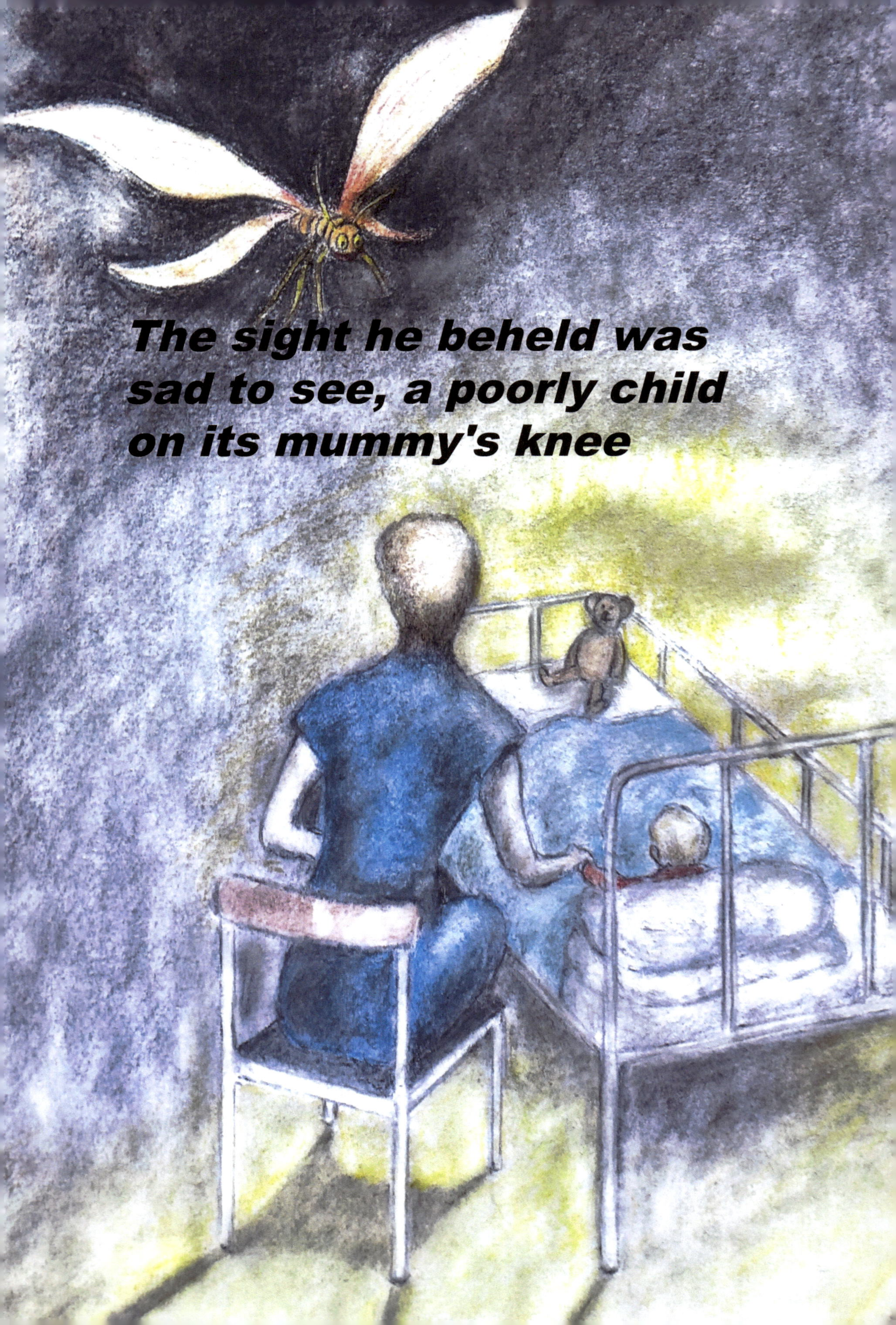
The sight he beheld was
sad to see, a poorly child
on its mummy's knee

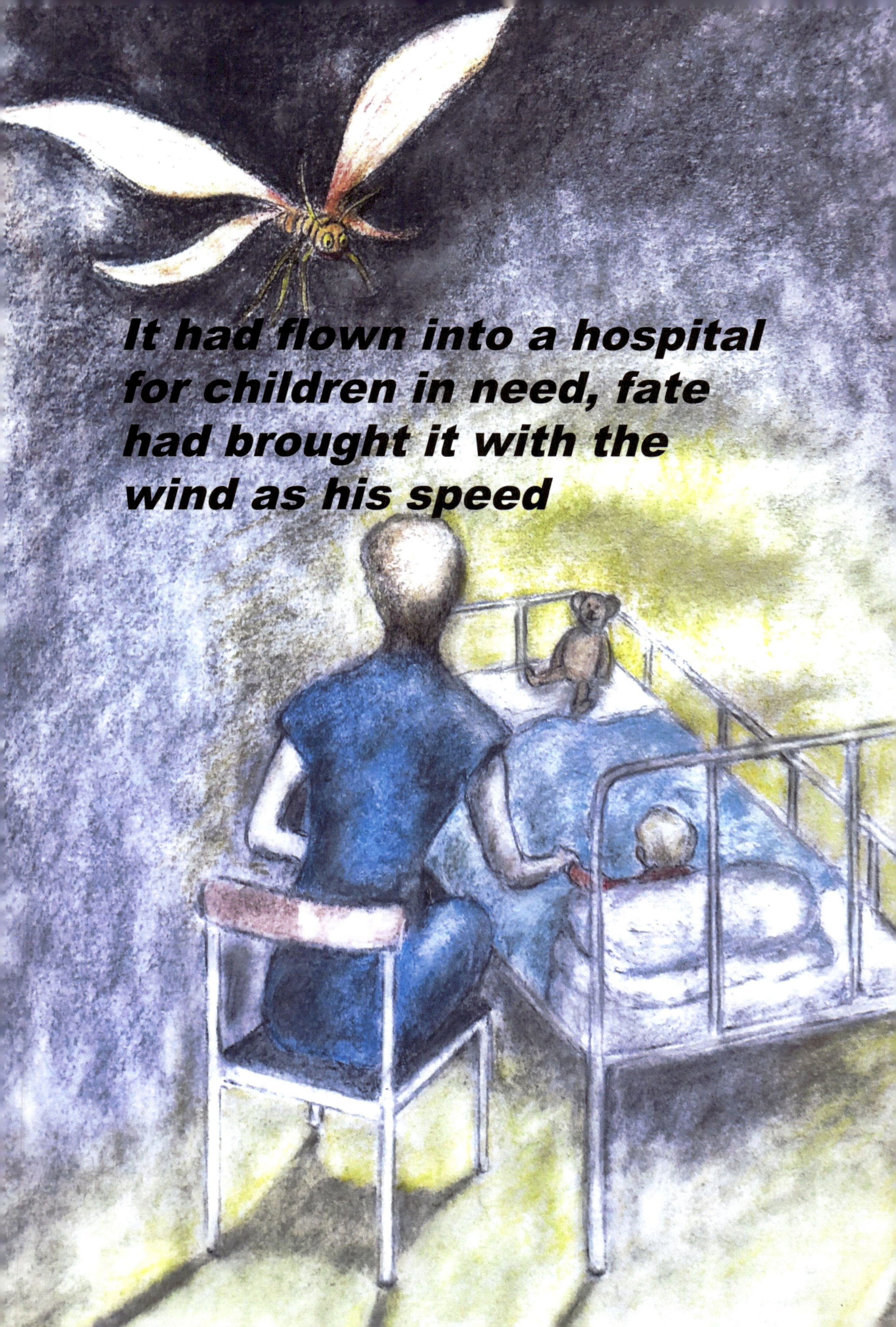
It had flown into a hospital
for children in need, fate
had brought it with the
wind as his speed

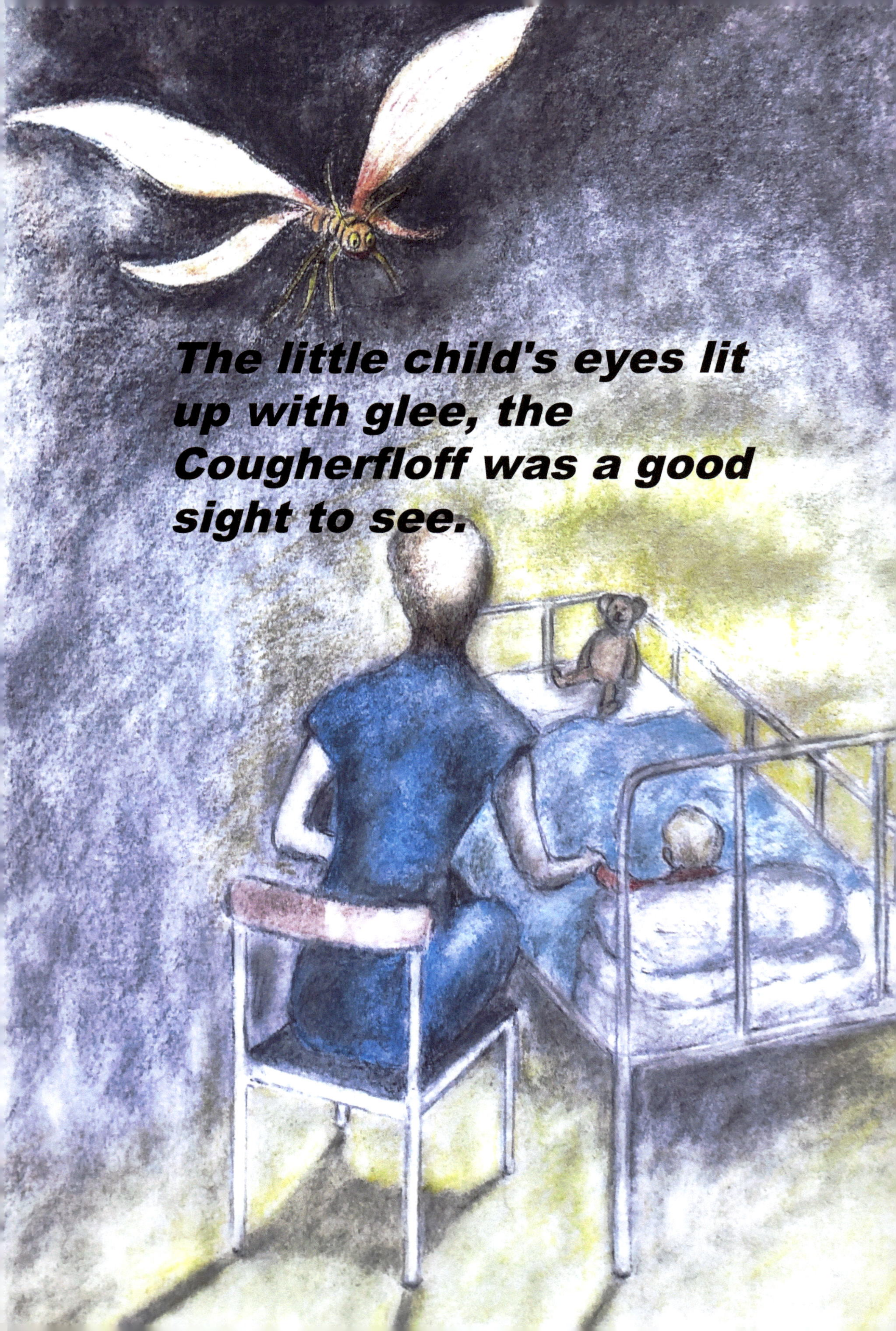
The little child's eyes lit up with glee, the Cougherfloff was a good sight to see.

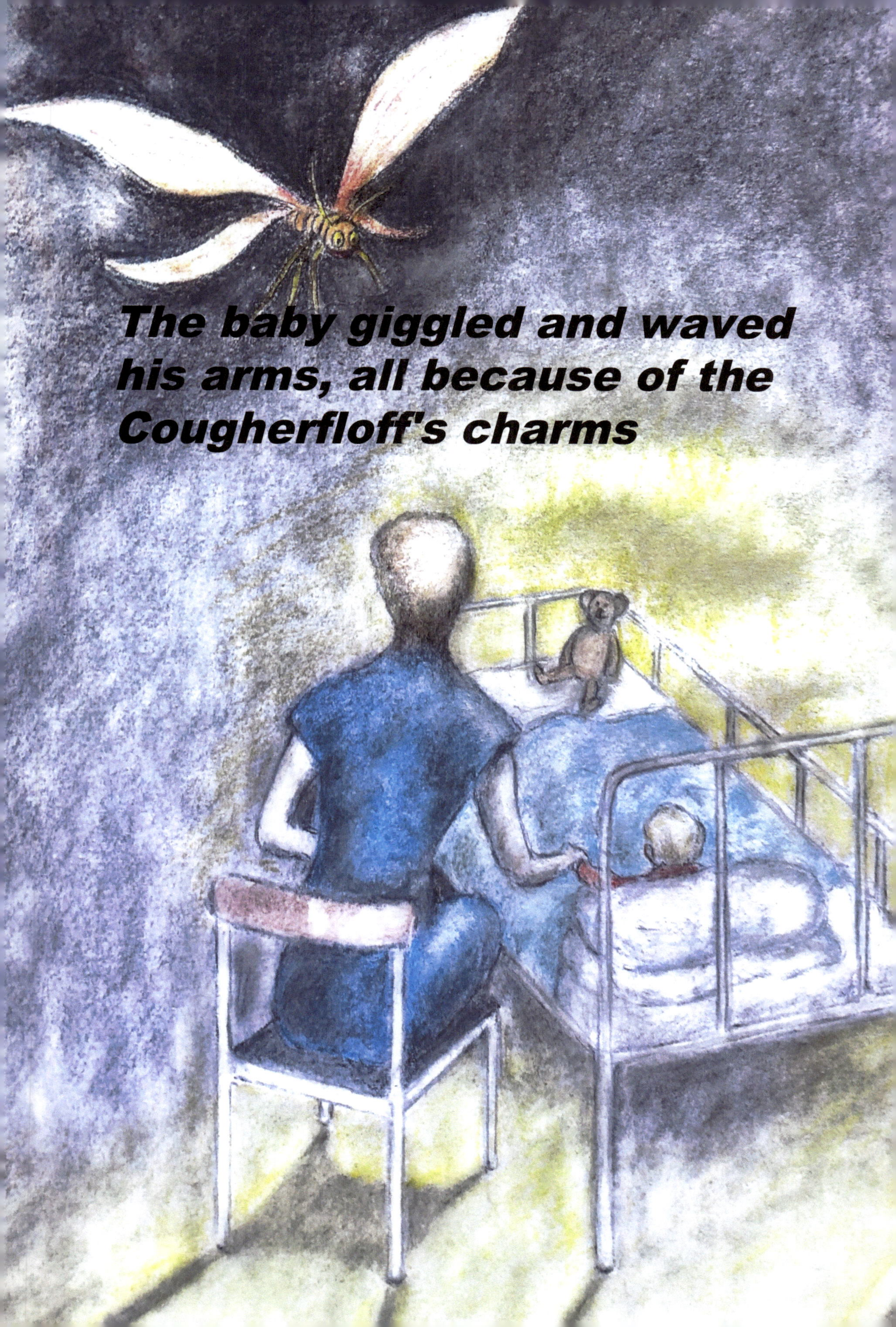
The baby giggled and waved
his arms, all because of the
Cougherfloff's charms

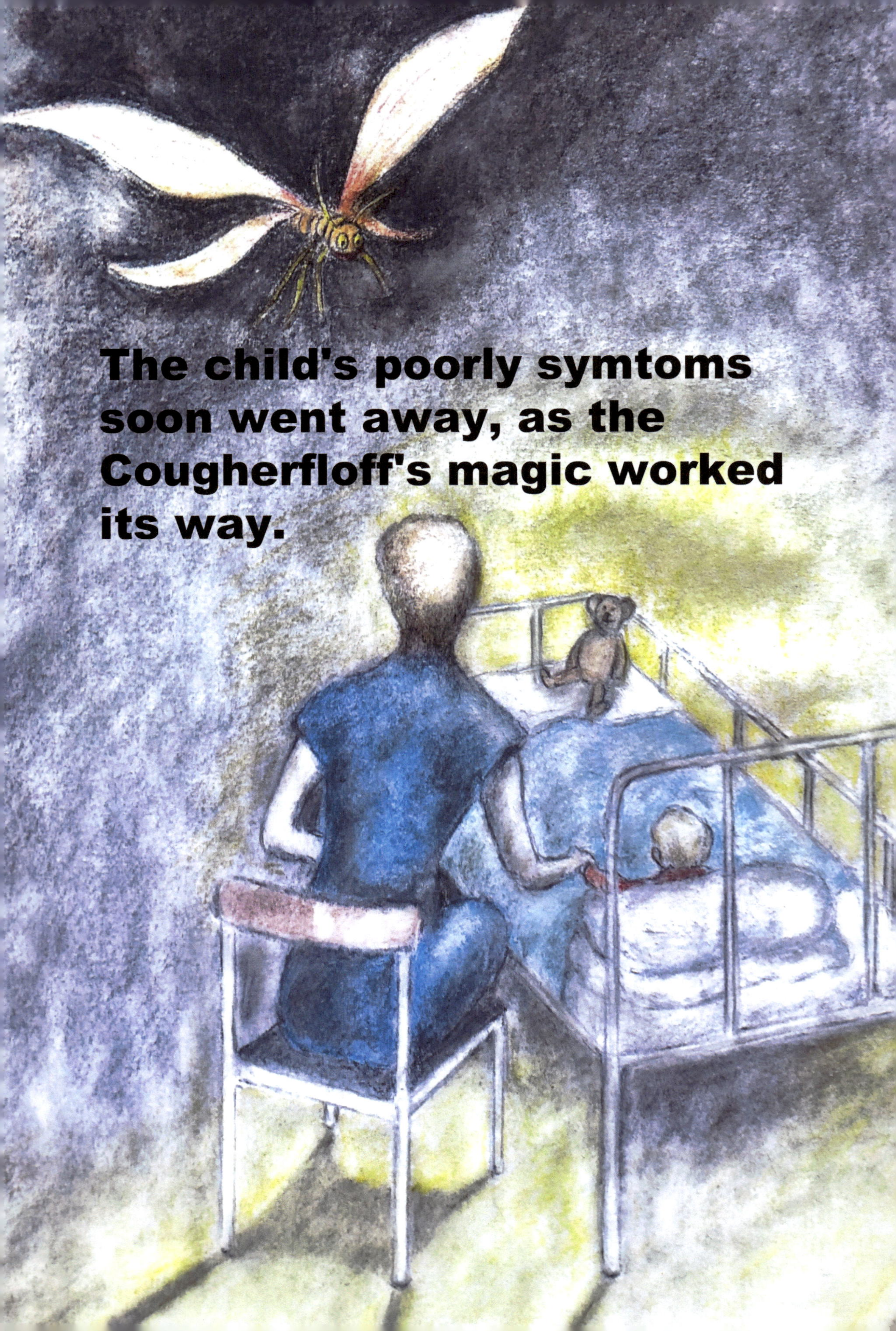
The child's poorly symtoms
soon went away, as the
Cougherfloff's magic worked
its way.

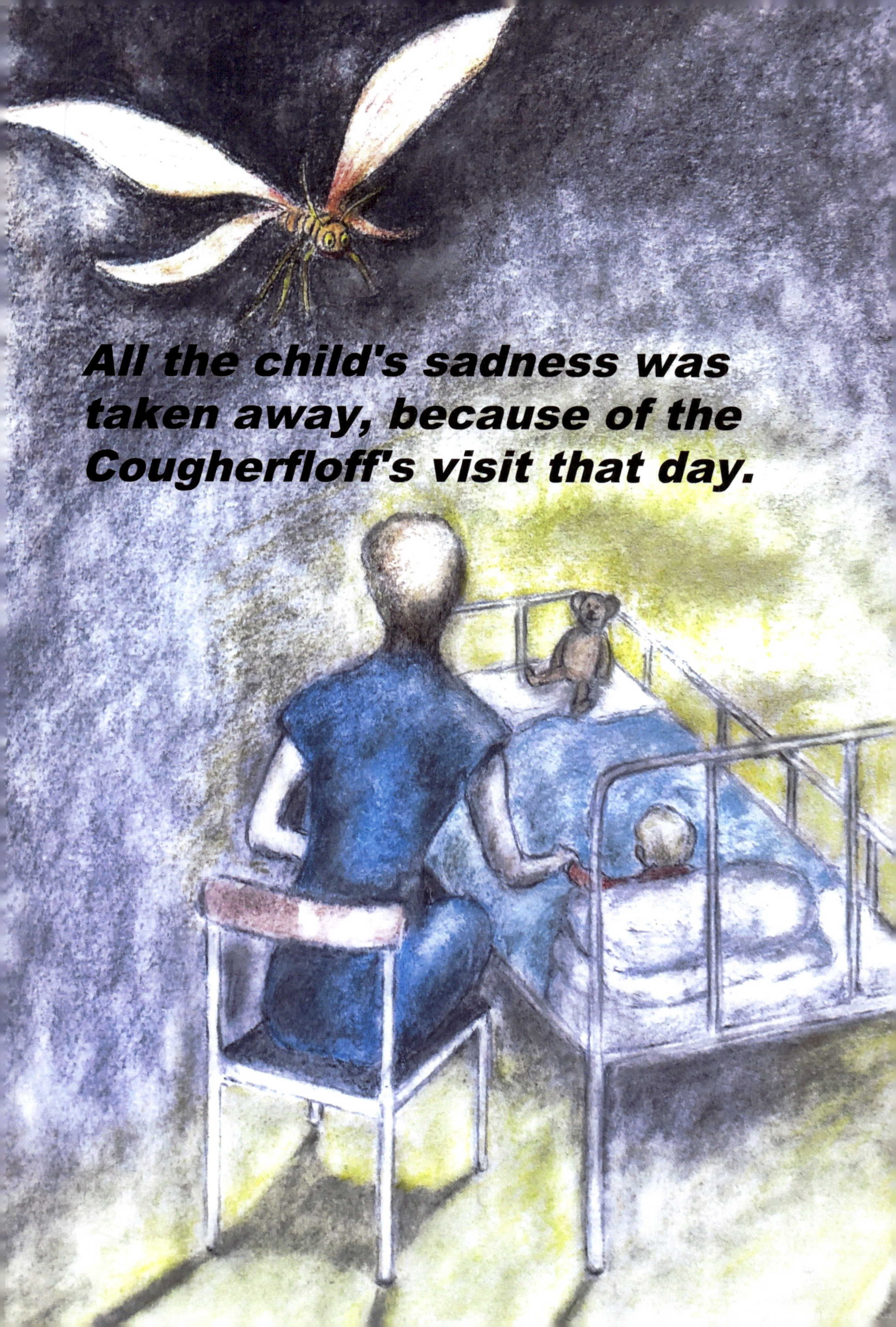
All the child's sadness was taken away, because of the Cougherfloff's visit that day.

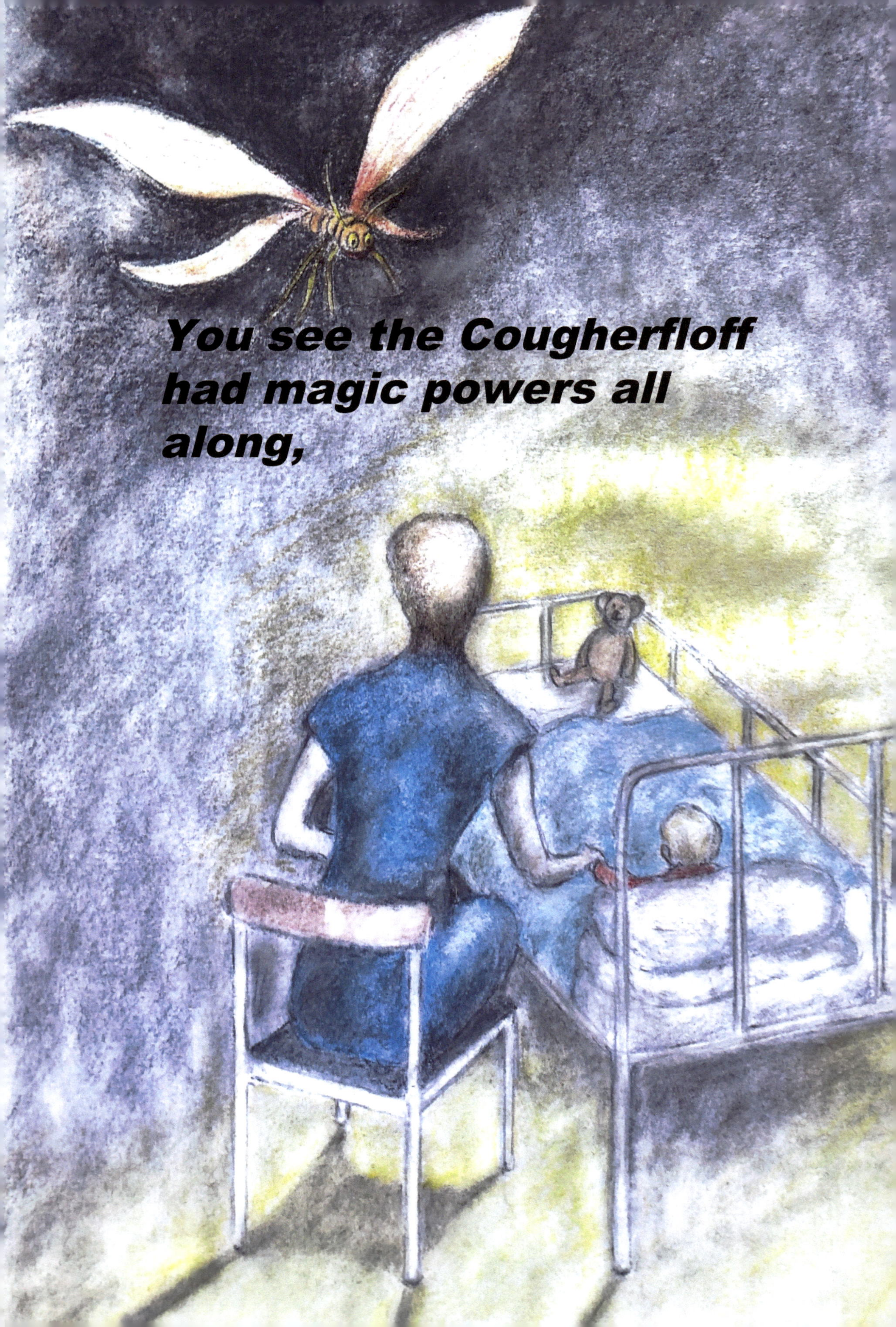
You see the Cougherfloff
had magic powers all
along,

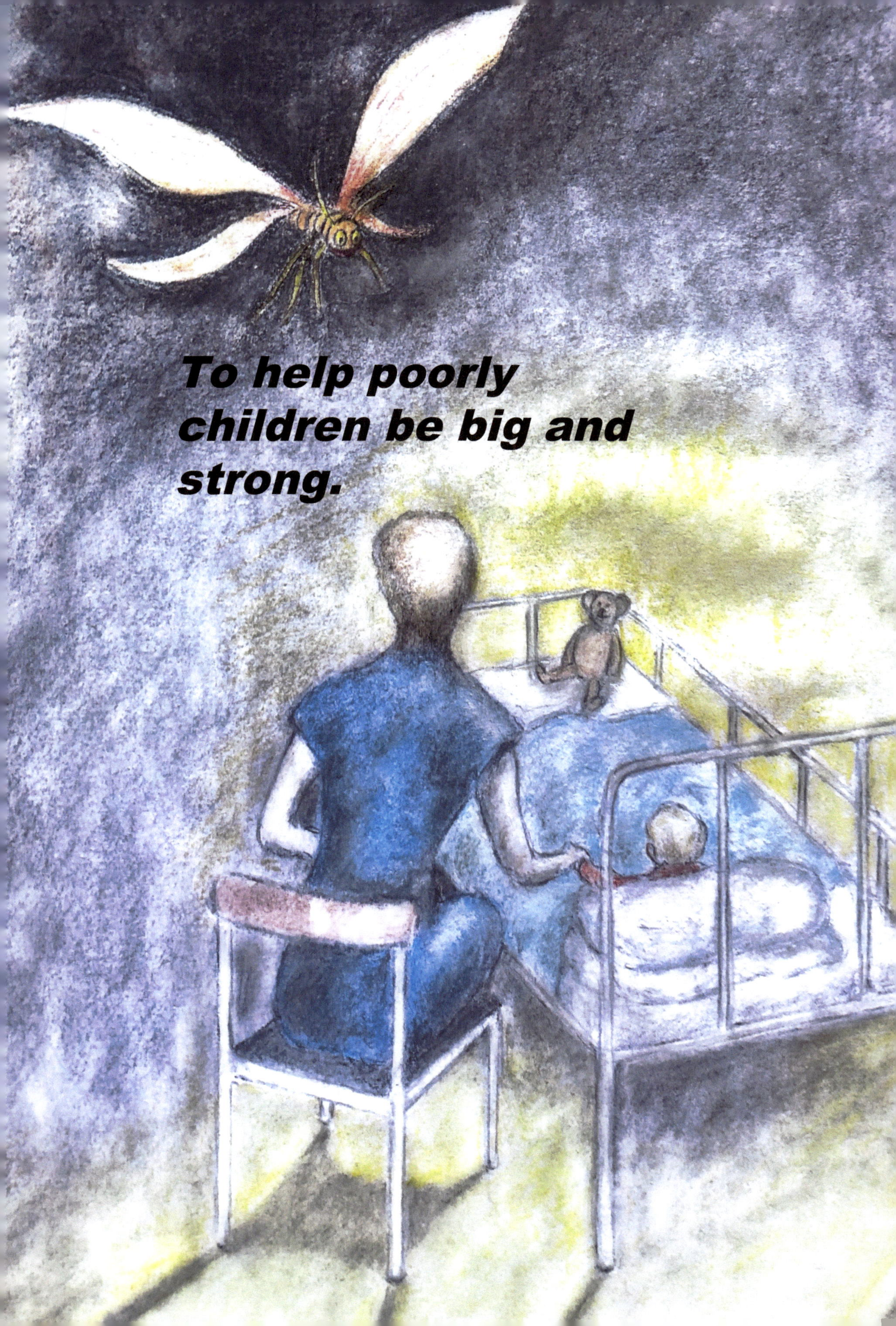
To help poorly
children be big and
strong.

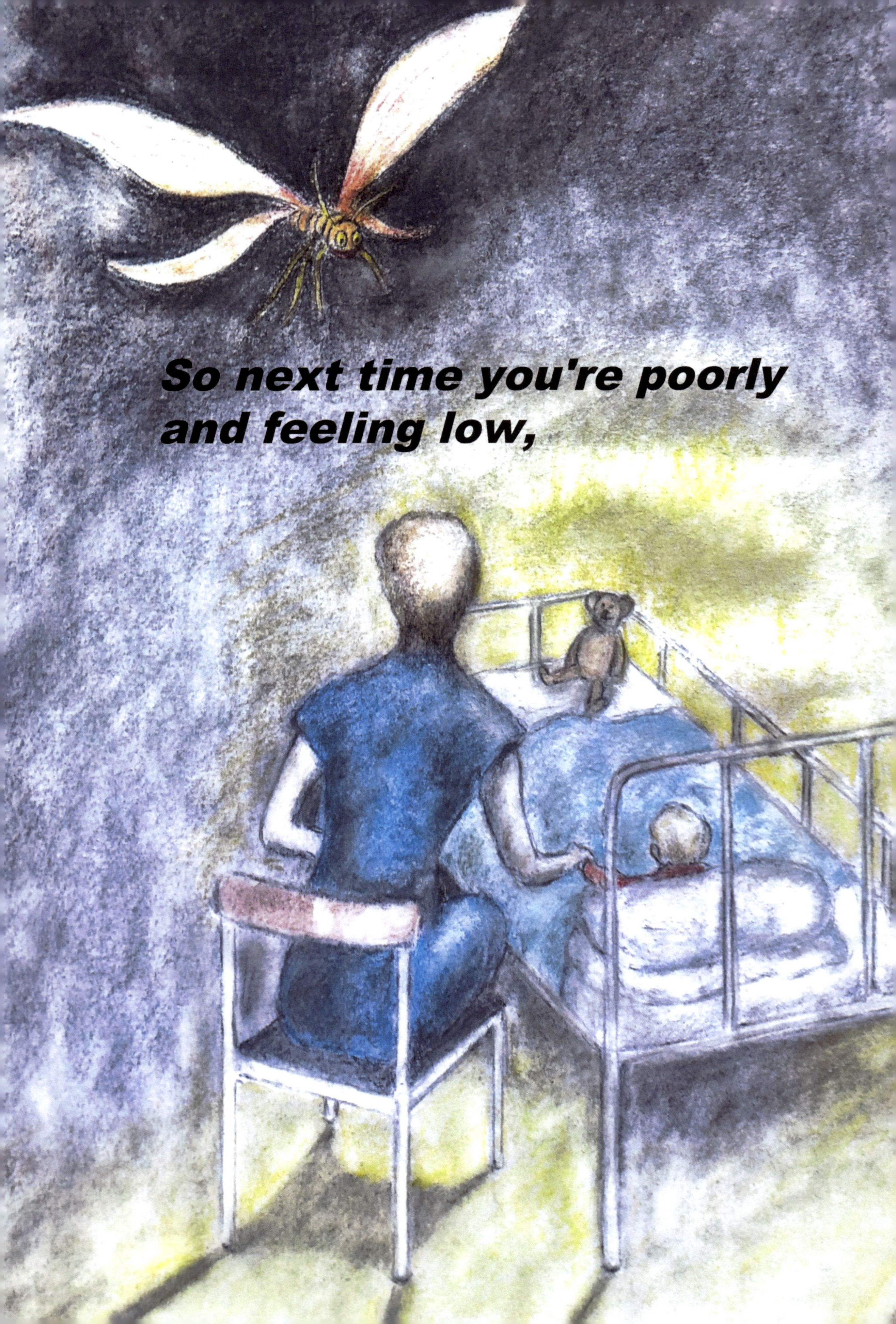
So next time you're poorly
and feeling low,

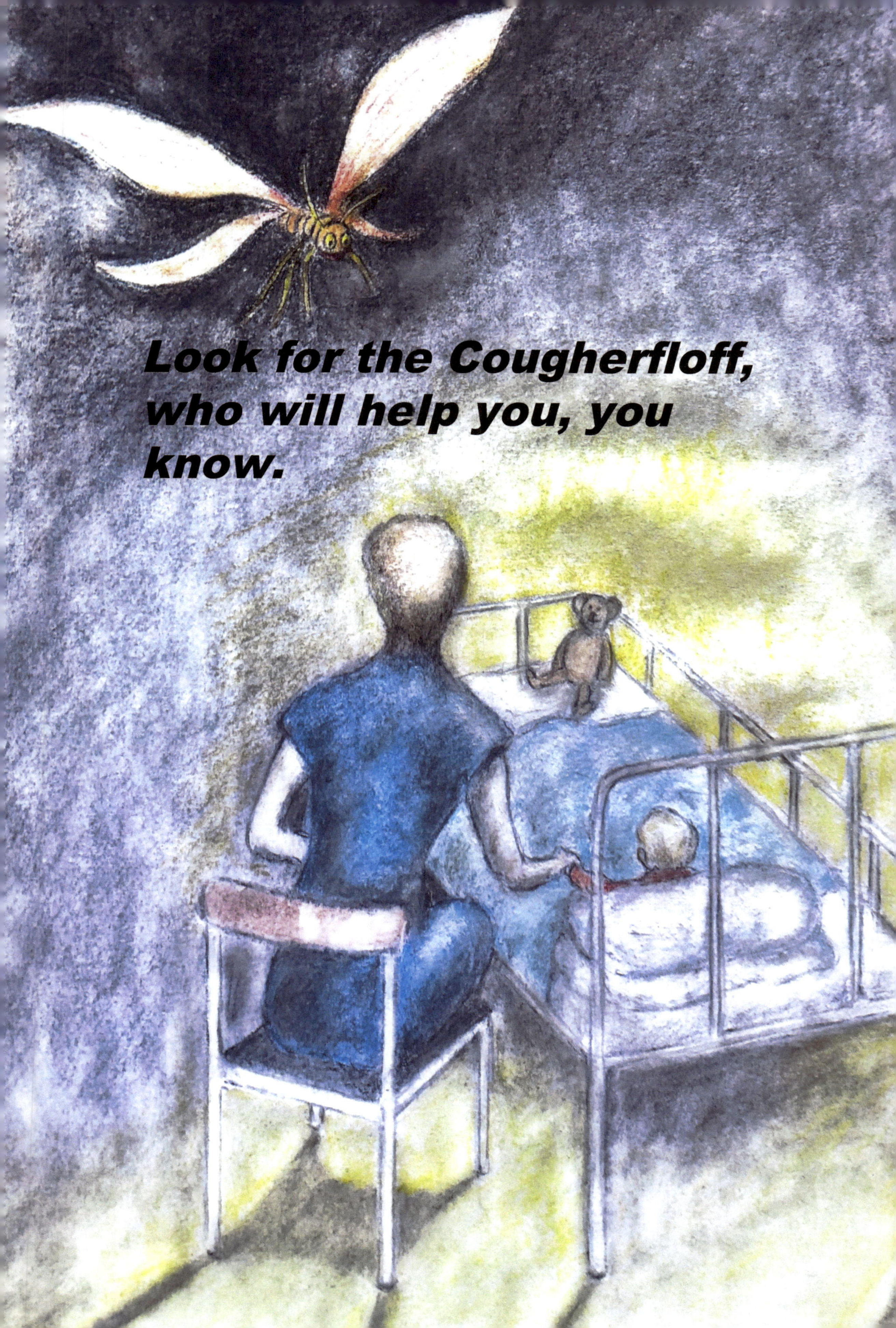

Look for the Cougherfloff,
who will help you, you
know.

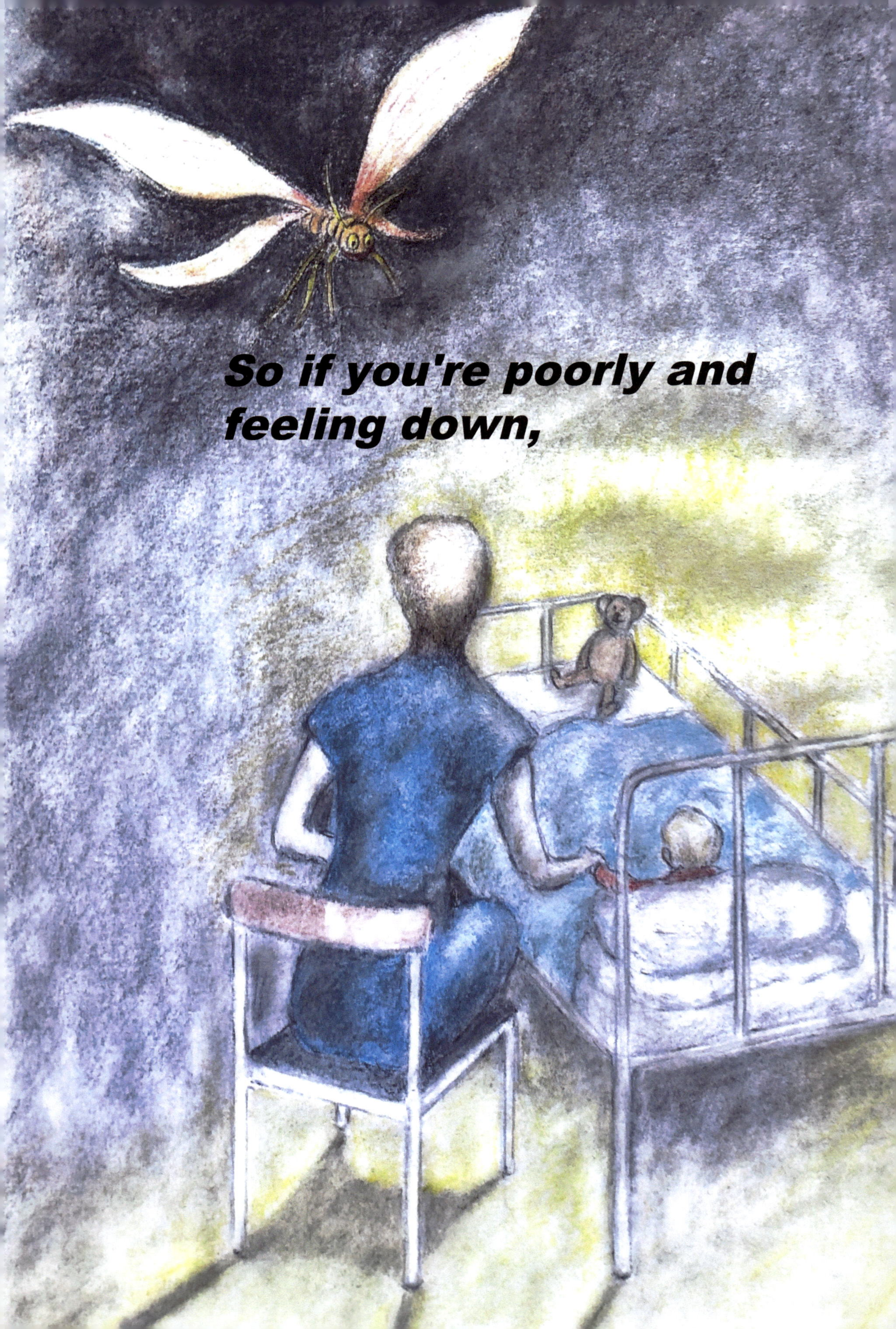
So if you're poorly and feeling down,

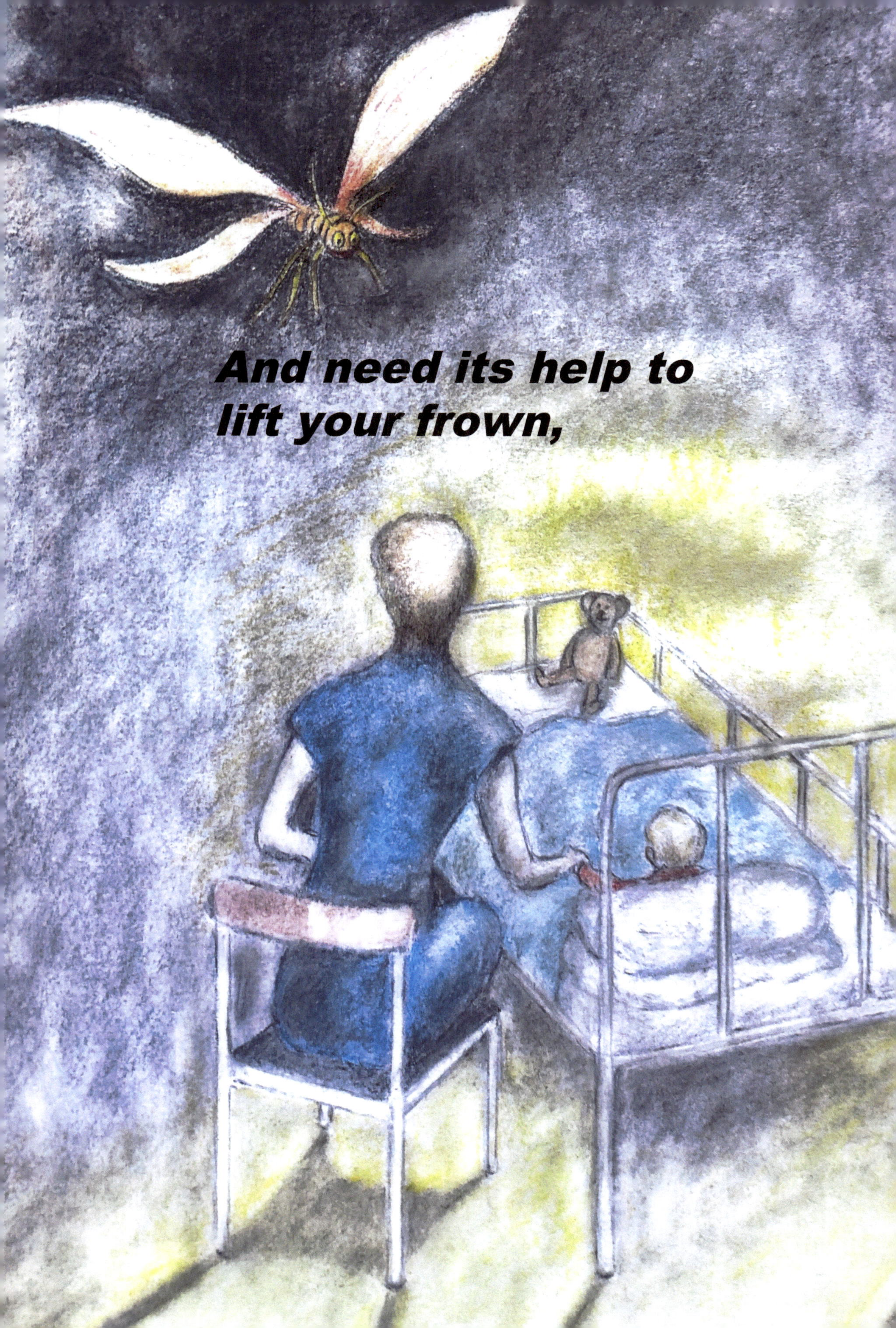
And need its help to
lift your frown,

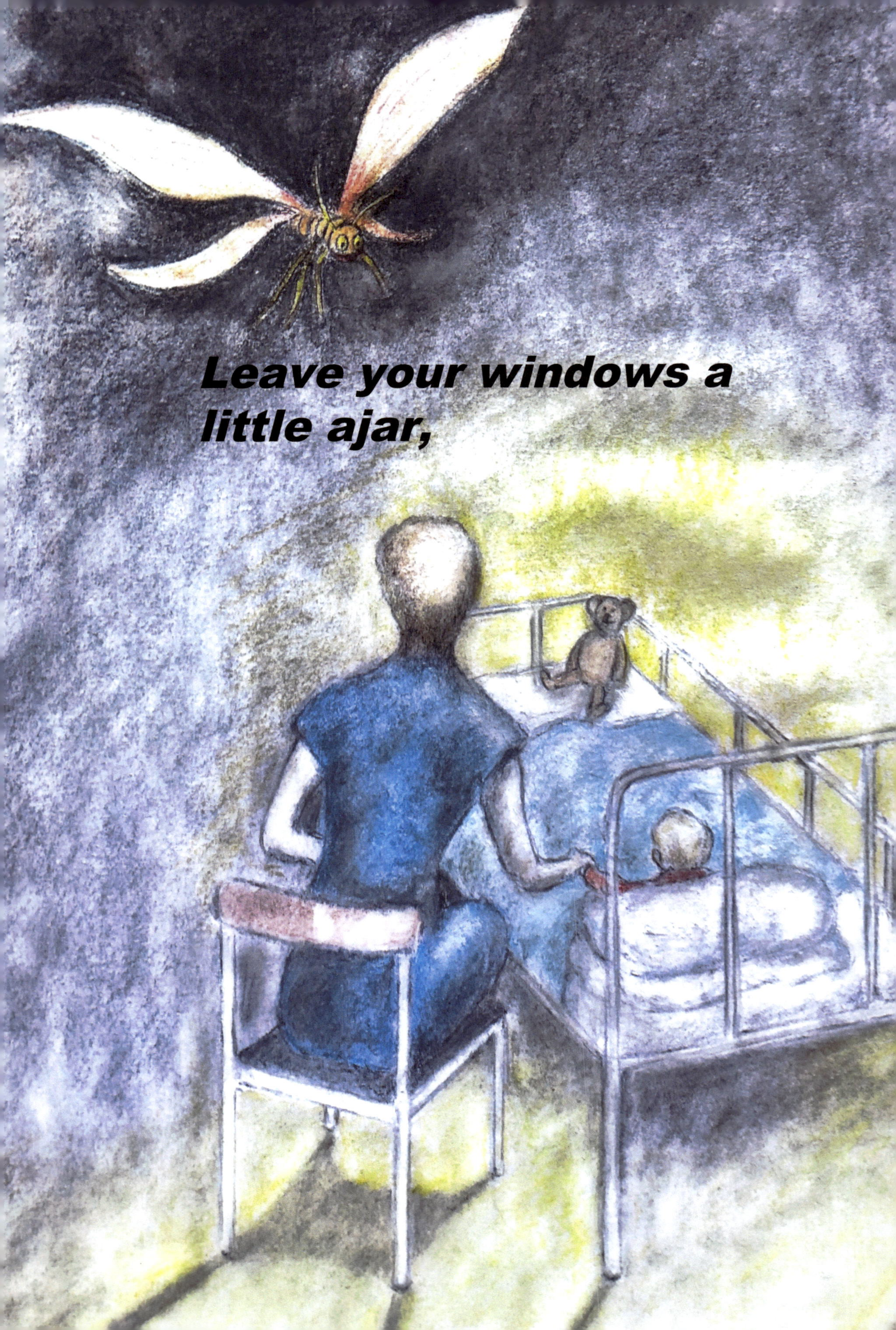

Leave your windows a little ajar,

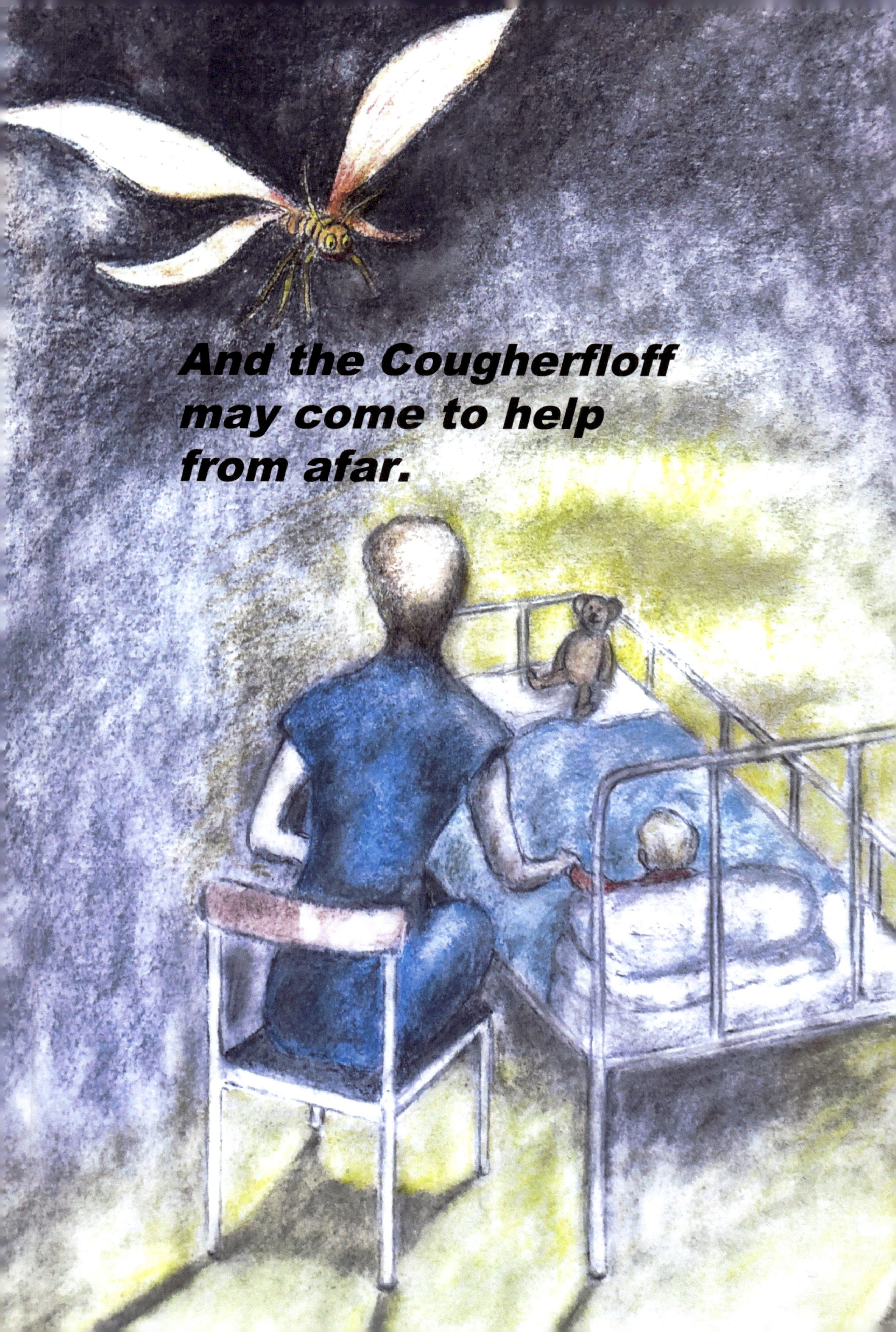
And the Cougherfloff
may come to help
from afar.

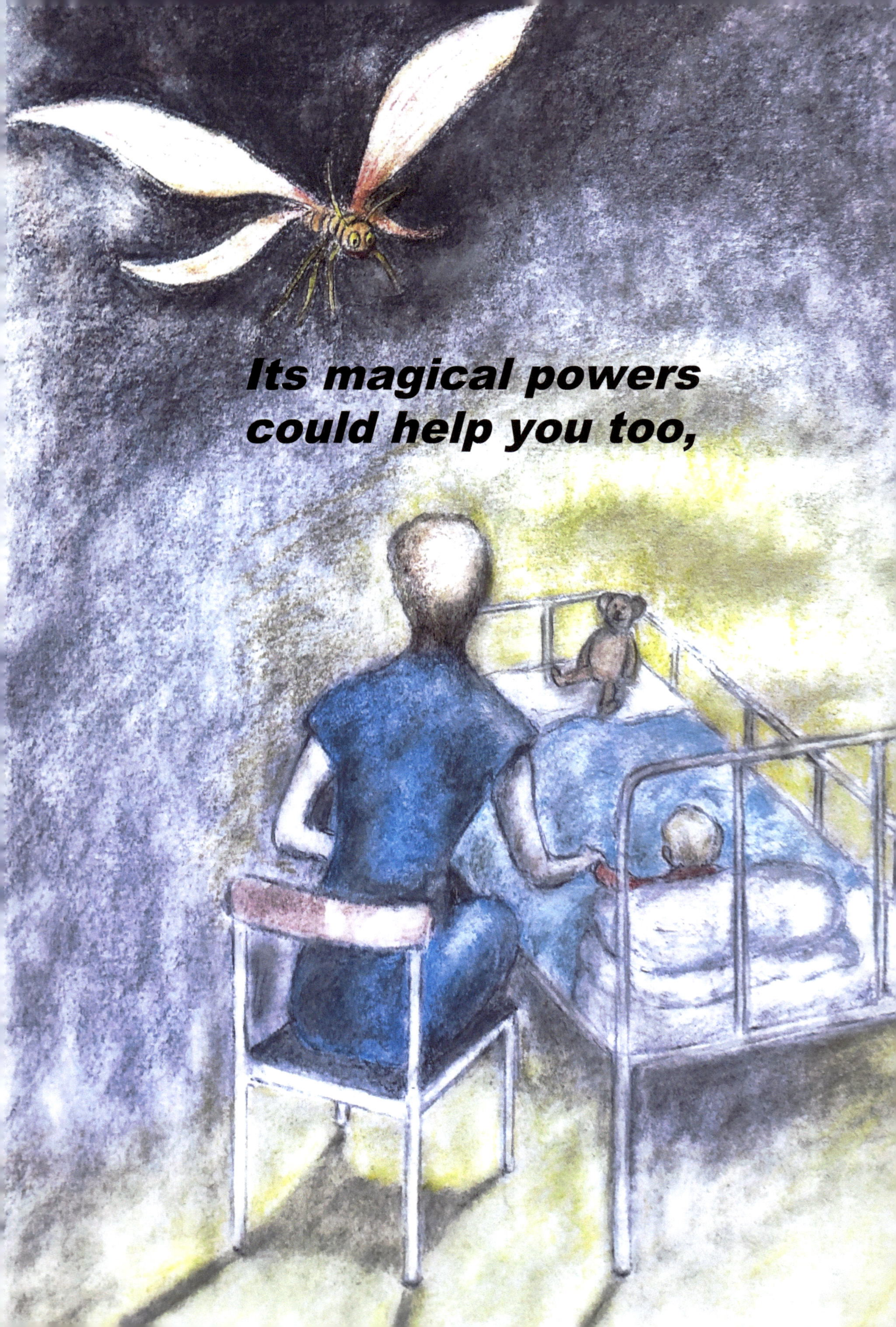

Its magical powers
could help you too,

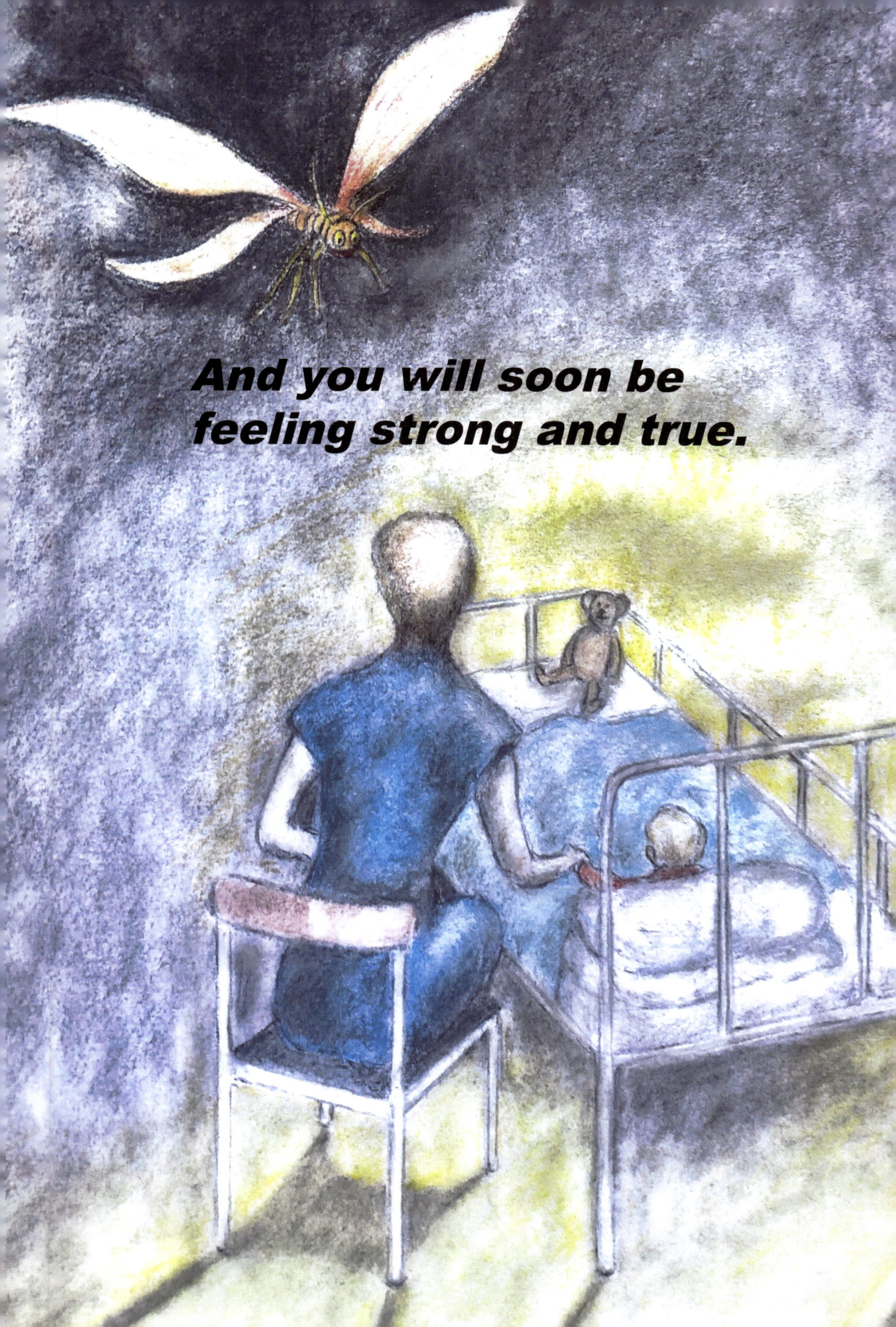

And you will soon be
feeling strong and true.

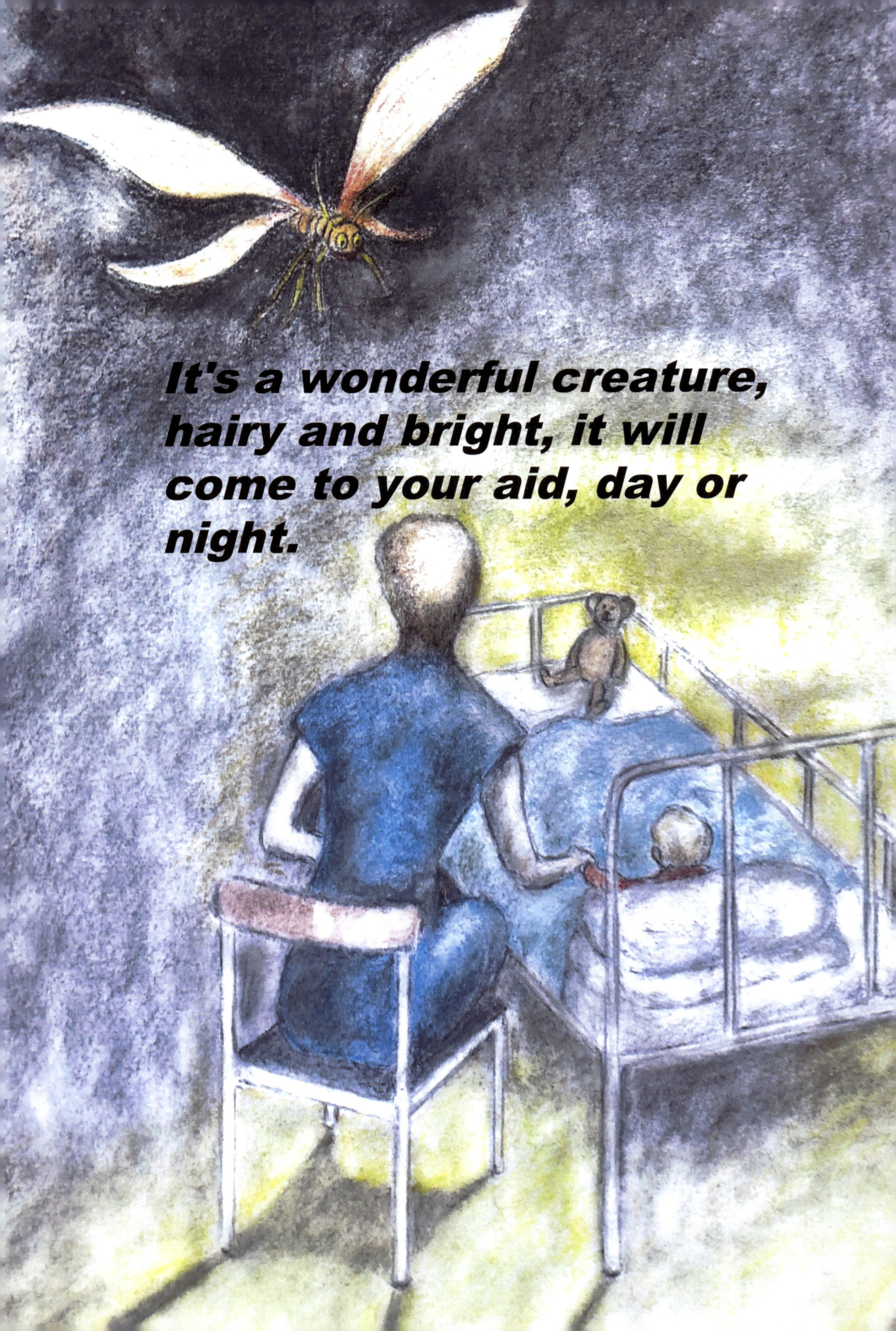
It's a wonderful creature,
hairy and bright, it will
come to your aid, day or
night.

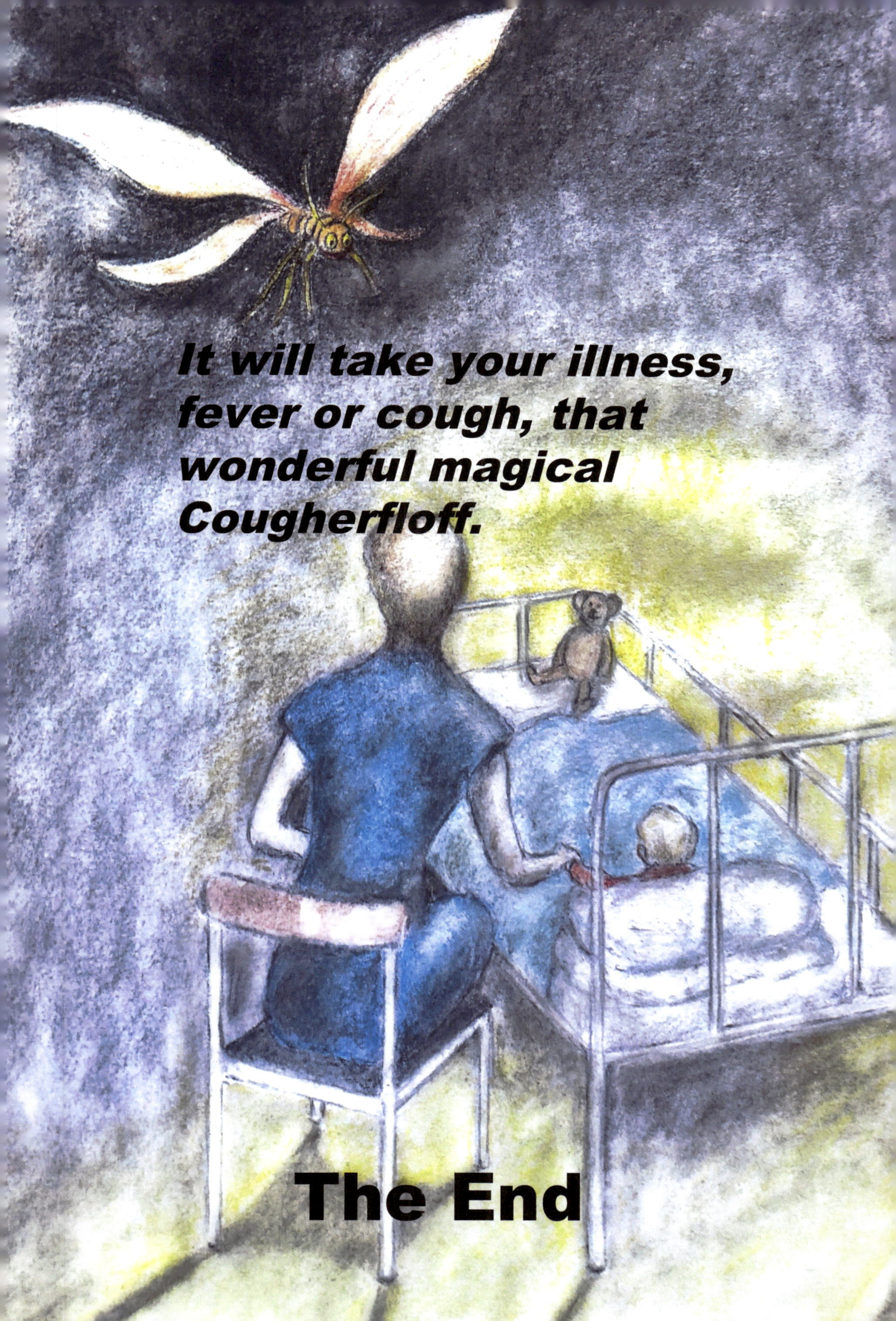

It will take your illness,
fever or cough, that
wonderful magical
Cougherfloff.

The End